5-DAY
TRAUMA WRITING TOOLKIT

A HEALING GUIDE TO TAKE YOU FROM PAIN TO PAGE

TIFFANY VAKILIAN

SPEAK FIRE
PUBLISHING

ISBNs

Print ISBN: 978-1-958978-37-5

Ebook ISBN: 978-1-958978-38-2

Library of Congress Control Number: 2025915484

This publication is designed to provide accurate and authoritative information in regard to the subject matter covered. Readers acknowledge that this work is sold with the understanding that neither the author nor the publisher is engaging in the rendering of legal, financial, medical, political, or professional advice. The content has been derived from various sources; consult with a professional when appropriate. Every attempt has been made to provide accurate, up to date and reliable complete information. While the publisher and author have used their best efforts in preparing this book, the advice and strategies contained herein may not be suitable for your situation. Neither the publisher nor the author shall be liable for any loss of profit or any other commercial damages, including but not limited to special, incidental, consequential, personal, or other damages.

CONTENTS

INTRODUCTION

Hi. My name is Tiffany Vakilian, and I am a trauma survivor.

It sounds so contrived and cliché. But if you've lived on this planet through 9/11 in the United States, you're a trauma survivor. If you've lived on through the COVID pandemic, you're a trauma survivor. Some are painfully aware, and some are blissfully unaware. But the truth of it is, those were traumatic times. We're in this together, having had these experiences. We are also survivors of the traumas specific to life experiences, locations, and choices.

I have seen, done, and had things done to me that have left indelible marks on my soul. The cool thing is, I feel truly and fully healed.

And here's why.

I went into that room—that deep, dark room of trauma—and I cleaned it out. Once I did, I knew my calling in life. I had to help others escape that room, so they, like me, could *go back into it*, look at it with new eyes, and realize what it could be.

That beautiful art of their life, that kintsugi,[1] was just waiting for them to put gold in it and remake the broken into beautiful.

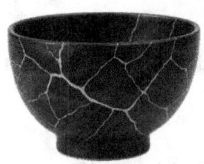

I knew from experience that, once they did that work, they would no longer have to label that room as the room full of trauma. They would have the freedom, power, permission, and choice to label it their own beautiful, bittersweet, soulful remembrance.

But it takes work.

This is not the kind of work where you put your hand to the plow and move dirt, or you drive to a location and sell something. You have to listen to your own voice, and let it tell you the truth.

You have to make your body, mind, soul, and space ready. If you're ready and willing, this book will help you create your space, overcome what's trying to stop you, keep yourself emotionally safe, and open the door to that room. Once do you, you can capture those details that set you free to see where your true self care needs are and how to move forward to write about that room, create that kintsugi, and set someone else free, just as you set yourself free.

---

1. kintsugi [*kin-tsoo-gee*]: Also called kintsukuroi [*kin-tsoo-koo-roi*]. a traditional Japanese pottery repair technique in which lacquer mixed with precious metals, especially gold, is used to fill cracks and replace missing pieces

This book is formatted and spaced out over five days to give you time for baby steps, but you can try do it in five minutes with this quick and powerful work.

Not only that. I will help you with:

- writing prompts

- a checklist for creating that very safe space for your writing

- self-care strategies for when you might need that extra time, space, and care.

Are you ready?
Let's get started.

Day 1

Creating Your Safe Writing Space

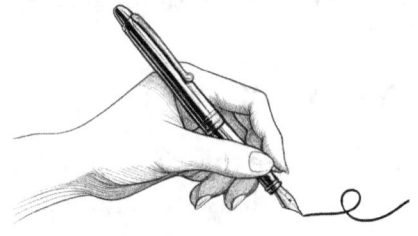

You've decided to want to want to. Day 1 is going to be the hardest work, but GOOD JOB. Day 1 may take days to do. Make space for that.

No really, make that space.

Be it mental, emotional, physical, financial, social, etc. It's important to give yourself room to think about the trauma you've experienced, let alone write about it. It's a pearl hidden in the clam of your protective measures. But if you're willing to dedicate space and time to your healing, you will find it in some form.

Yes.

You.

Will.

Did you know that, if you create a dedicated space for yourself, that space can help support your emotional regulation. I want that.

I want that for you, just like I want that for me. I *need* that for myself. Every day, triggers try and get my heart racing, head throbbing (or worse, fuzzy), and my plans stalled. How about you?

Satan doesn't need to take years, he only needs to take seconds or minutes, and if I am not careful (with dedicated space for dealing with these battles), I will give hours, days, weeks, months, and years away. If you've ever felt that, then lets try and get you some dedicated space.

The (Mostly) Physical Space

Your writing space is more than just a physical location; it's the crucible where your ideas take shape.[1] Try to identify a quiet, private area in your home where you can make room for calm breathing, meditation, or prayer...and writing. If space is not available (or only available in small quantities), you can find a way to create the space. You can buy or make room dividers. You can convert a space to serve multiple purposes. A lot of moms with small kids have said their bathroom is sometimes their only sanctuary. If that works for you, great! But maybe it's your car?

Sometimes, you have to go outside. Perhaps there is no physical space where you are. So "where you are" needs an imagination overlay. And sometimes, you don't have time to get to the mancave, she-shed, bathroom, bedroom, car, wherever.

Guess what?

For a short period of time, you can close your eyes and go to an imagined place. It is a solution. Trust me, hiding in the bathroom is a true respite at times, and not just for moms.

---

1. Heres's a cool website I found about creating a writing haven: https://at mospherepress.com/optimizing-your-writing-environment/

But eventually, you will have to honor yourself enough to move things around. You still have to set up the space.

Set Up Your (Trauma-Informed) Stronghold

Real or imagined, you need to make the space work for you. Let's pretend your space is a room in the mental house that represents you. If you can go into that physical space right now and start the shift, that's great. But for now, let's act as if we're working on our room in our house. You need to ask yourself some questions

What are your seating options?

Make sure they are comfortable, because your body needs to relax into that space so you can "start the art" of kintsugi for your soul. You'll need more than one seat for yourself. Yes. More than one seat (though I admit, the floor is always the second chair). Make the chairs (couch, loveseat, beanbag, mound of pillows, etc.) as fluffy and floofy and designed the way YOU want and need. Those chairs are going to hold you as you work through the room of your trauma.

Should you ever decide to allow someone into that space, they must adapt to your special space. This space is made by you, for you. There is power in that.

How's the light in there?

You **NEED** light!

The antithesis to the dark disease of trauma is the light of the witness, and that is you.

You are the one to tell the story, to uncover the truth, the reveal "the real" to yourself, and share your safely unsealed heart with others. **You are the witness.**

That light can be found, no matter how dark the times seem to be. The sun comes up every morning, even on cloudy days. And clouds won't block the sun forever. Proper lighting is natural, and it adjusts.

Consider the "lamps" you have in there, so consider the hue of the light. Think about its warmth and versatility because that comfort helps you to focus for more writing. You are setting yourself free, make that space do the heavy lifting.

Temperature control

Your space has a temperature is relatively controlled by you. It may be a hand fan, an electric fan, an air conditioner, heater, multiple blankets, fuzzy socks, that one cardigan that grandma gave you. You are not uncomfortable in that space because you've taken steps to cover your skin with the cool, heat, cover, breeze. It is your space, and it should calm your soul just as it gives you room to breathe.

There, you will inhale peace and exhale your kintsugi writings.

Sensory-Friendly Places and Spaces

There are many, many books about the psychological need to make your space calm and clean. It sets the stage for you to be able to pour out properly. Not only that, having your space clear of unnecessary clutter will do one major bit of heavy lifting, because it gives space within your space for you to hear your own voice.

For those of you who have, or are currently working with a licensed, clinical professional, make it a point to note their space. See how it serves your calm, and what they do to change when it doesn't. Someone who knows and studies the need for calming environments makes it a point to create a calming environment and to become a calming influence as a human being. Why don't you take a moment and think about sometimes when you felt calm and what was going on around you? What were the colors? What were the senses that you felt on your hand? What did you see Had you just eaten? What were you eating? These are the kinds of questions you can ask yourself. when you start thinking about your sensory experiences. so that you can incorporate them into your space.

Minimizer potential triggers

Your relaxation is a battlefield where triggers are constantly trying to take ground. Don't leave the enemy's tools in your space.

One of the ways you can minimize potential triggers is to try and learn what your triggers are so you can deny them access to your space. Simple spaces tend to remove potential triggers, as well as make your brain connect that space with writing and writing work. We want that. Use natural elements make your body "embody" the natural desire to relax and release.

Here are some other options you can use to calm the voices and open the heart to create:

- Incorporating calming scents (many people use lavender, vanilla, and I prefer Egyptian musk and woodsy scents like cedarwood and amber)

- Bringing in soft, comforting textures (as I said earlier, blankets, cushions, and things like that)

- Selecting soothing background sounds or music

- Visual elements for focus or inspiration (I love books, plants, artwork) Check out my office book-shelf:

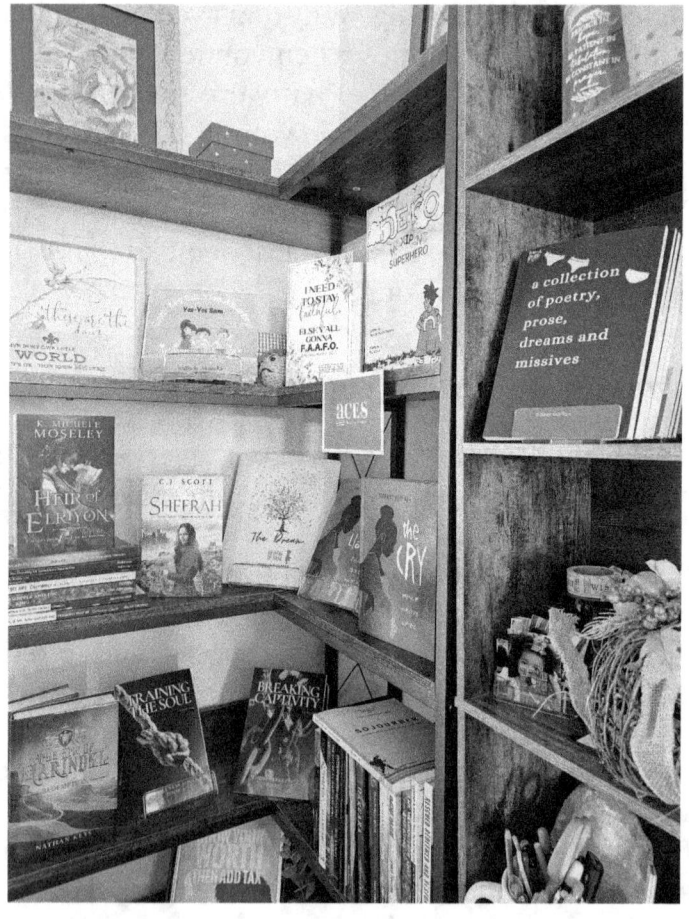

This is my pride wall (of books I've either edited or published), and I've specifically ordered these books to look at them for inspiration, focus, and because the covers are pretty. I also move them around for fresh perspective.

Writing Tools

I have edited books that have been digitally written and physically written. It's easier to edit the digital copy because the fonts are easier to read, especially when you have a very enthusiastic writer. But that doesn't mean that you need to pick one or the other. You can use both. Whichever one will help you get the story out is the one you need. So pick the one that will serve your freedom, peace, and joy.

And guess what?

The device might change depending on the trauma!

No matter what, though, you've got to keep the appropriate supplies nearby. So for example, if I'm using my computer to type, I make sure my keyboard works for me. I like having a mechanical keyboard because I like the clicky sounds. However, I am a mother of two, so I also use voice-to-text, which has saved me quite a bit of time. Not only that, speaking into a recorder is a part of my dual expression coaching.

You might also want to have a special journal for writing about your particular story. Ish you are using digital tools and perhaps a folder would best serve, or a special name for the file. You could even use a totally different app. just so that you tell your brain we're working on this. When you're done, you can close it up and walk away, keeping it separate from the day to day things. Sometimes the stary needs to be locked away, prepared for engagement, engaged, and then left alone.

Your emotional safety is the most important things here.

Emotional Safety Tools

As I write this, I'm dealing with a death in the family and an active Flare-up of Small Intestine Bacterial Overgrowth (SIBO). I am reeling on multiple fronts during a traumatic response, and I am fully overwhelmed. Not only that, I am not home. Remember the beautiful space that I created just for me? I am nowhere near it, so I am here to tell you these tools can be created on the fly if you are able to recognize the possibilities.

Create a Grounding Kit

Do yourself a favor and keep a grounding kit nearby or on you (like a fidget keychain or soothing pebble). For example, keep journals in various locations, along with pretty color calligraphy pens. That does it for me. For others, that could be a stress ball, a fidget ring, a fidget spinner, a certain pair of shoes or other comfortable clothing, etc.

Do what works *for you.*

But don't be afraid to explore other options that you haven't considered before. They might work for you as well. I saw a grounding kit on Etsy (no, I don't have the affiliate link), and it addresses the five senses. If those items don't work, then I will reach out to someone who's outside my situation, or at least more removed from it than I am at the moment, and I will ask them to provide support (sometimes just by holding space in silence). It's a good idea to keep an emergency contact list of people who are equipped to listen to you.

Go to (or Create) a Comforting Environment

Sometimes you just need to comfort yourself by creating or going to a space that is truly enveloping with good feelings and good vibes.

- You can go to a coffee shop if you like the smell of coffee.

- You can go to the beach if you like the sound of the ocean.

- You can take a walk if you live in a neighborhood that is suitable for that.

- You can read your favorite book.

- You can look at a photo that brings you joy.

These are all perfectly acceptable, and they will help you to prepare for that writing time, just as I am doing right now, as I create emotional safety and creative space for myself in real time.

This brings me to my next point, which is setting boundaries for your writing space.

Set Boundaries for Your Writing Space

I know it sounds strange, but it actually is a excellent idea for you to create ground rules for your writing time and space. There are plenty of ways that you can structure your writing time, including using Pomodoro timers or attractive, musical timers on YouTube.

For instance, tell yourself, "I will take 5 minutes to write about..." and then you pick your topic and you write.

It's a good idea to communicate boundaries to your family or your household members that you are in your writing space and you're taking your writing time. And they will need to respect that by giving you space and time. You can even create a ritual for entering and exiting your creative writing mindset. Using these tools, even if it's only for 2 minutes, will give you a greater sense of peace about what you're about to do regarding writing about your trauma.

Additionally, you will be able to leave it more easily because of the sense of ritual that has a beginning, middle, and end.

Grounding Exercises

One form of ritual, as I mentioned before, is beginning with some grounding exercises. Here are a few:

- 5-4-3-2-1! This is a sensory awareness exercise where you pick an amount (five through one) and assign it to one of the five senses. Five things you hear, four things you see, three things you taste, etc.

- You can never go wrong with any form of deep breathing exercise. You can make it specific to your space, and it can help you outside of the writing space as well.

- Getting in touch with your body by stretching is another effective way to prepare yourself for writing, and honor your space with your embodied emotions.

Practical Exercise – Create a Checklist

Create a checklist for your writing space set up.

1. How is your space?

2. Can you move your space? Do it "go with you?"

3. Is it friendly to your sensory adjustment? Does it give you peace, calmness, inspiration? Do you feel safe there?

4. Do you have a ritual (of any type) that helps you access your mental writing space?

What about you? Do you have any other questions? Feel free to grab a journal and add questions, or other checklist items that work for you!

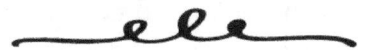

Day 2

Getting Started: Baby Steps and Self-doubt

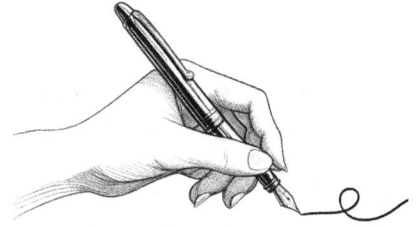

Writing Day 1 took me weeks to complete, because I was living the book as I was writing it. One of the major battles I faced was the one I had with self doubt. The word for day 2 is GRACE. Today we are going to put pen to paper, or finger to keyboard, crayon to parchment...we are going to write.

It's going to be okay. We are going to babystep the whole thing.

But first, we need to face something kinda sucky, which is addressing self doubt and it's blocking abilities. Like I said, today is about small forward moment. Totally acheivable stuff, if you are ready. We are going to take those baby steps, after we deal with the elephant in the room. This is a hard battle, but small bits of faith in yourself, to just move the pen, to just type *one* word, all add up to something wonderful and freeing.

Address Self-doubt

Day 1 was so important, because there are plenty of tools listed, but I have some more for your toolkit!

Here is a list of effective strategies for addressing and overcoming self-doubt (I'm not defining them, I am just listing them. If I defined them, we'd stay in that rabbit hole and not do the work needed here):

- Practice Self-Compassion

- Remember Past Achievements

- Reframe Your Thoughts

- Set Clear Goals and Make a Plan

- Surround Yourself with Supportive People

- Practice Positive Self-Talk

- Adopt a Growth Mindset

- Keep a Journal

- Take Action Despite Doubts

- Seek Professional Help if Needed

This list is not exhaustive, and I did dive deep into some of them during Day 1. But just know you can do this, you can write, and you are worth the work.

The other day, I found myself listening to the rustling of an aging palm tree in the wind. For that moment, I was calm, focused, and "okay."

That moment with the palm tree grounded me, gave me a sense of peace, and was so memorable that I wanted to share it with you. I will use that moment to give you a freewriting exercise.[1]

Freewriting

This is one form of pre-writing, which I think is an important way to "prime the pump" before you get into the details of your own lived experience. Freewriting is something you can do on by writing on paper with a pen or pencil, using a keyboard or stylus on an electronic device, or even using a recording device to transcribe your thoughts. I did some freewriting about that tree, and though it has been months, I can think about it and go right back to that place. Every time I think about how grounded, safe, and free I felt, it retrains neural pathways, tracing and strengthening my brain, which heals me physically, mentally, and emotionally.

That is the power of freewriting, so here is a freewriting offering for you:

> Take a moment and imagine yourself standing a few feet from a lone palm tree. It's tall, healthy, but a bit older. The dying palms hang down, shaking gently in the wind. What do you hear? See? Smell? Feel? Taste? Take five minutes, and journal about that.

---

1. Freewriting means a writer doesn't stop writing and doesn't take the time to edit or adjust the ideas on the page even if a mistake is made. From https://www.uis.edu/learning-hub/writing-resources/handouts/learning-hub/freewriting

Stream-of-consciousness Writing

Stream of consciousness is a narrative style that tries to capture a character's thought process in a realistic way... includes a lot of free association, looping repetitions, sensory observations...

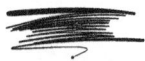

...and strange (or even nonexistent) punctuation and syntax...Thought isn't linear, these authors point out; we don't really think in logical, well-organized, or even complete sentences.[2]

Let's try the "Lone Palm" prompt again.

Take a moment and imagine yourself standing a few feet from a lone palm tree. It's tall, healthy, but a bit older. The dying palms hang down, shaking gently in the wind. What do you hear? See? Smell? Feel? Taste? Take five minutes, and journal about that.

This time, don't edit yourself. If your brain goes on a tangent, let it. Follow that thought wherever it will go, and after five minutes, stop and look at (or read) the art you made.

Practical Exercise – Let's Write!

Using either Stream-of-consciousness or Freewriting, do
two or three exercises (give yourself about three minutes
for each exercise). Allow yourself the freedom to pause, or
to write, what is really coming out of you.

Day 3

Distancing Techniques for Emotional Safety

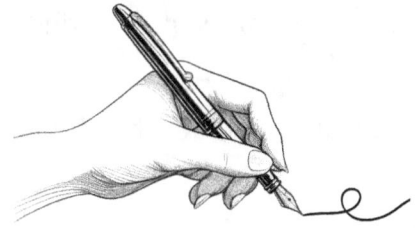

Feel free to go back to Day 1 and Day 2 as many times as you need for reminders. Today, we're going to explore the door and the front three feet of "the room" you are going into. Here are some pointers for entering, standing there, leaving, and writing about your experience. Try one, or all, of these options at once. Some folks need time for each step. Honor that. You can also find more that are specific to you, and add them here. You are worth finding and using the unique things that make you healthy and whole!

Write in Third Person

First person perspective means that you are living the experience with all of it's weight. You use the pronoun, "I" when you would talk about something that's happening.

This can be traumatizing when you're dealing with that room. But one way to buffer yourself is to use the 3rd person perspective, saying "he," "she," or "they." This puts some mental distance between you and the experience, even if you are the person you are talking about. For example, you can say:

I went to the store and bought some tacos.

That's first person. 3rd person is writing it like this:

She went to the store and bought some tacos.

Do you see how responsibility is placed on another person, mentally taking the brunt of weight of so it is no longer on you? This is a great buffer and might work every time. But there are other options.

Use Metaphors and Symbols

Not that I am trying to give you a crash course in light English, but a simile compares something by using the terms "like" or "as" to make the connection. A metaphor just connects one thing to another. For example,

The yellow dress she wore made her look like a taco.

The phrase a simile because it uses the word "like."

A metaphor would say it like this:

She was a taco in that yellow dress.

When I'm writing about trauma, I tend to use trees. Right now, I am not even in a place where I can even go into the room. But I have a feeling that I will be writing about forests in the not-too-distant future.

Change Perspective

This pocket guide[1] I found online has quite a few awesome ideas, and it gives an awesome description of changing perspective:

> [Write] from a new, unexpected perspective—maybe not as the person who's lived through the trauma, but as the grown child of the victim. Or a passerby who glimpsed what happened. Or a tree that has lived for decades on the spot near a crime.

I love their reference to a tree. I think that it is rather powerful to have found that description as I was working on today's chapter. I don't take those kinds of coincidences lightly, and I am grateful. By even taking this moment, I am transforming myself for the better, reaffirming my good memories, and making stronger ties to them than to the "the room."

---

1. From: https://www.spreadtheword.org.uk/a-pocket-guide-to-writing-th rough-trauma

Once again, there are other options for you to try for distancing techniques, but for the sake of keeping both you the reader, and me, the writer, from overwhelming ourselves and losing focus, I'll stop here. If you know of any, or feel the need to research more tips, tricks and hacks, please use them. Don't limit yourself. I know I won't!

Practical Exercise – About "That Door"

Using one of these distancing techniques, or one you find/create on your own, write for three minutes about the "door to that room."

When you're done, take a moment to breathe. You're doing hard work, and it is not without honor. I honor you work, and I honor you.

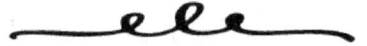

Day 4

Capturing Sensory Details

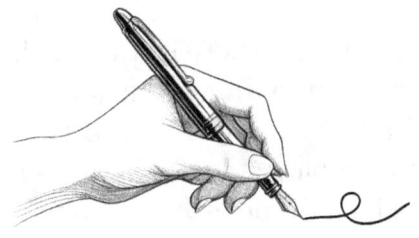

Days 1 through 3 are done and you're still here. Thank you for not giving up. Let's go back to yesterday's writing (if you feel ready to do that. You can also just write something new). Today we are going to rewrite that mini-manuscript. I pray that the rewrite makes it easier for you to view. If not, give yourself the grace to know that you don't have to. Write something else to work on!

Today we are going to work on three rewriting perspectives so that you can exploring breakthrough experiences and lay that beautiful gold over the story.

Focus on the Five Senses

As I've said before, what happens in the five senses can actually ground you, calm you down, and work peace through you at a cellular level.

Why wouldn't you want to write through those lenses? Embody the five senses through the pen, keyboard, or voice recorder? Use your five senses to review what you've written about and expand it to include those details because those details are vital to you—and any other reader who sees your work.

Describe Physical Sensations

Similar to using the five senses, it is a great idea to describe the physical sensations of things that are going on. If you're sitting in a chair, perhaps you want to talk about how the fabric feels, or how hard it is. Perhaps you tell the reader about how high it is off the ground and what your feet are doing.

Ask yourself, as you are writing about this particular detail, how does this feel in my body? Combining the five senses and the physical sensations really brings the writing to life. The more you unpack, the more you unload. And even if you burn this work after you write it. Set it all out there when you set it on fire!

Right now, I'm sitting in my chair and my tailbone is a little sore because I've been sitting for a long time (that is its own story). As I write, I could explain the pressure in my tailbone. The discomfort is trying to take my focus. My hurt is not completely unbearable, but it's a definite a mild bit of pain.

I can pull the reader in to that detail within a scene.

You can do the same with writing those kinds of details within your own space.

Avoid Premature "Meaning-making"

I'm sure you've heard the phrase, "everything happens for a reason," but I think it's really important that we don't shortchange your traumatic process, even as you write.

If you aren't on the other side of the thing, then **that's okay**. If you still need time away from that situation, **that is OK!**

When you try to find reasons or meaning before you process, it is like having knee surgery and trying to sprint two days later. When you do this, it dishonors your beautiful story and silences your voice within your lived experience.

Please, please please please DO NOT DISCOUNT WHAT YOU HAVE BEEN THROUGH. Mourn the way you need to, because it is your journey, your story, your kintsugi.

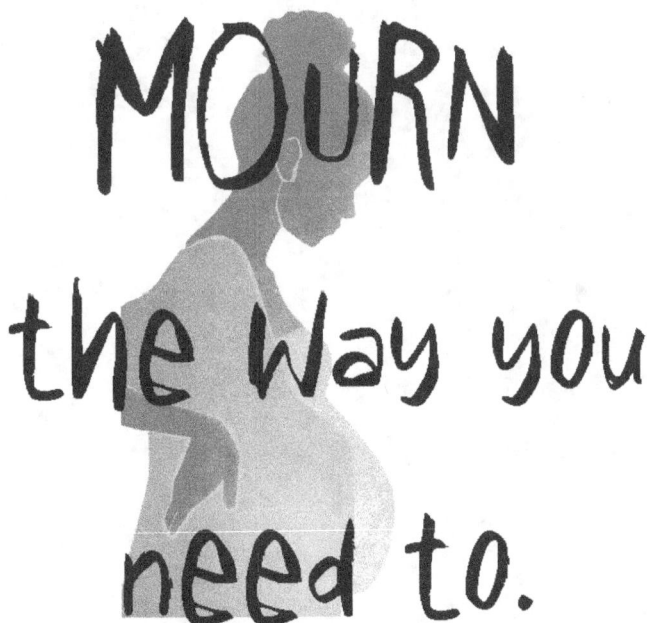

Practical Exercise – Kintsugi Bowl Edit

Rewrite your scene (or, if you're feeling brave, write a new scene). Try using one or more of these sensory capturing details. Try doubling the length of your piece, or if you need a wordcount, push for 300-500 words or more. If you typed or used voice-recording technology, why don't you try for 500-750 words.

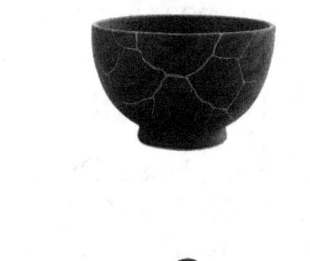

Day 5

Moving Forward and Making Time for Both Writing and Self-care

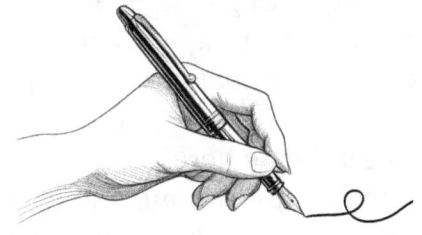

I have tried my best to be open, honest, and intentional about giving you grace and space throughout this writing journey. It's only been five days, but I think a lot of you are going to take so much longer than that.

GOOD FOR YOU.

Take that time and space.

I would rather you be healthy than writing, because I know that if you are healthy, your writing will be more powerful.

And now you're on Day 5. Hopefully you've looked at day one repeatedly to remind yourself of the different ways and spaces that you need. I hope you've worked on Day 2, opening up the door with baby steps to writing. I hope you've taken time for consideration of Day 3, to make space for your perspective to remain healthy.

I hope you did the Day 4 work, expanding your writing.

Now we're on Day 5, making time to grow from here, both on the page and in your self.

Set a Manageable Writing Pace

If you start with a ritual of five minutes a day, as long as you're consistent. I'm okay if you do a two-minute ritual, as long as you're consistent. If you have the time and the space to make an hour long writing once a week, great. If you can do a monthly writing weekend getaway writing, great! Whatever you do, make sure that you can be consistent.

Are you sensing a theme here?

I don't want you to do too much and then burnout. I also don't want you to do too little and not experience the true freedom and healing that is available to you through writing.

Breaks will happen. Life will go on and interrupt your schedule. Make it manageable, so you can take breaks as needed.

Post-writing Relaxation

Speaking of breaks, it's a great idea for you to do a post-writing relaxation at the end of the day or at the end of the writing (even if it's for only five minutes). Anytime you go near "that room," you need to give your body a chance to process it out. Sometimes what is physically going on as you process your writings can be your body processing emotional poisoning.

You've got to make room for that because if you don't, it could work against you.

I've personally experienced somatic releases of emotional toxins in the form of muscle spasms, headaches, back aches, and things of that nature.[1]

So, at the end of your writing, take a few deep breaths. Give yourself a statement (some may call it a mantra) to let you know that this process is over until the next time. Close the loop and leave it until the next time. This is a way to honor your writing, your processes, and schedule. You are worth the work.

Make sure that you take yourself so you can finish your story. One way to do that is to reach. outside of your mind or home to your local people

Connect with Support Systems

Support systems are not just for trauma overload. However, those special friends who are able to hold space for you and make you feel seen when you are having a trauma response are worth their weight in gold.

Connecting with support systems can be as simple as going to your favorite coffeehouse or tea shop (Hey there, Bliss) and saying hi to *your* regulars. It could be going for a walk in the park and seeing the same people. One really notable place for support is church. If you have church friends or groups that you spend time with regularly, they can offer support on the daily pragmatics of life, not just for when you're processing trauma.

Once you start recognizing your lanes, you can create a strong framework for healing, writing support and self-care.

---

1. https://www.news-medical.net/health/Somatization-Symptoms.aspx

When you are really rocking and rolling through the writing, you can really unlock a lot of gems that can help you heal and grow.

Practical Exercise – List Your Groups

It's a good idea for you to have a ready-made list of people you can turn to in a pinch, whether it's for pragmatic stuff or for traumatic stuff. Make a list of things you can do, places you can go, and people you can talk to, both for the day in, day out life minutiae, as well as for the trauma. If you can, you can skip writing it down, but I do NOT recommend it, unless your brain is really good at holding that data (even under pressure).

Do not forget phone numbers for licensed professional (local numbers or even the national hotlines).

You are art, and your story is worth having this kind of support.

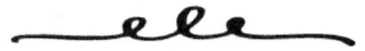

Bonus

Writing Prompts, Safe Space Checklist, and References

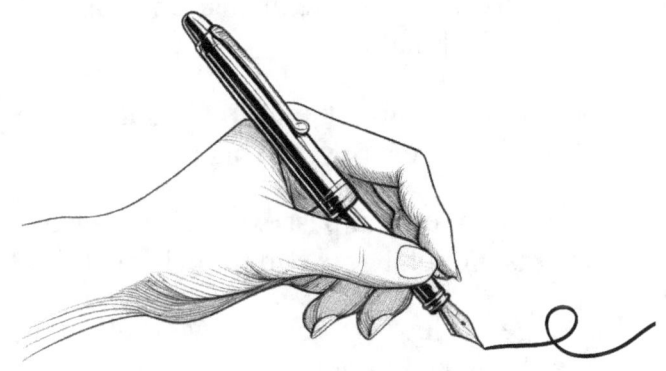

10 Writing Prompts for Starting this Process

1. Write about your current emotions without judgment. How are you feeling right now as you begin this journey?

2. Who in your life makes you feel safe enough to be vulnerable? What qualities do they possess?

3. When did you first realize what happened to you was trauma? If you didn't recognize it at the time, what made you understand it later?

4. List five people, places, or things that make you feel completely safe and take three minutes for each person to write an explanation about why they make you feel that way.

5. Describe the strongest emotion about your experience as if it were a physical place.

6. How do you feel your past experiences have shaped your present behaviors and thought patterns?

7. Write a gentle letter to your younger self about what you wish they had known or heard at the time.

8. Write a letter to your body talking about how you physically respond when you think about your experiences.

9. What strategies have you developed to feel safe in your daily life? Which ones help and which might need adjustment?

10. Write about one small step you can take to show yourself kindness and begin healing.

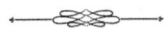

Checklist for Creating Your First Safe Writing Space

- Choose a private location where you won't be interrupted or actively observed by others while writing.

- Position yourself where you can see exits/entrances to help maintain a sense of safety and control of your environment.

- Set up physical comfort elements like a supportive chair, good lighting, and proper writing gear to avoid bodily strain.

- Put comforting objects nearby that can help you feel grounded.

- Place grounding objects within reach - something with texture to touch if you need to reconnect with the present moment.

- Create a list emergency comfort contacts (trusted friend, therapist) easily accessible if you need support during your writing.

- Provide yourself some gentle boundaries by turning off phone notifications and letting others know this is your private time.

- Have soothing items accessible - tissues, water, tea, or anything else that helps you feel cared for.

- Keep a dedicated notebook or journal that feels inviting and safe to write in.

- Password-protect your digital writing files to ensure your words remain private until you choose to share them.

- If your items are not digital, have a place where you can secure them so they remain private until you decide they no longer need to be.

- Make yourself a small pre-writing ritual, like lighting a candle or taking three deep breaths, to signal this is protected time.

- Conversely, make yourself an exit ritual to signal the end of the process.

Modify this space as needed. You will change, so this space will need to change, too.

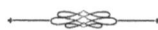

Self-care strategies for emotional regulation

Physical Comfort Strategies

Create a **comfort kit** nearby while writing that includes a soft blanket or comforting texture, something soothing to drink like tea or water, something soft to wipe any tears away, and a grounding object for holding or having nearby.

Emotional Safety Practices

- Set a timer for writing sessions with built-in breaks to prevent emotional overwhelm.

- Start and end each writing session with a calming ritual like deep breathing or a brief meditation.

- Write only in a private, comfortable location where you feel secure and won't be interrupted.

Grounding Methods

- Take short walks or do gentle stretching between writing sessions to release physical tension.

- Keep soothing music playing softly in the background or use calming scents.

- Have a trusted friend or support person "on call" during writing sessions.

Recovery Tools

- Give yourself permission (without judgment) to stop writing if emotions become too intense.

- Have specific coping activities ready for after writing - like listening to uplifting music or cuddling with a pet.

- End each writing session by noting three simple things you appreciate about your present life.

Remember to honor your pace! You have to go at your pace, and that includes stopping. Breaks happen. Honor them as a part of your healing.

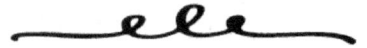

DUAL EXPRESSION™ AS A TOOL FOR YOU

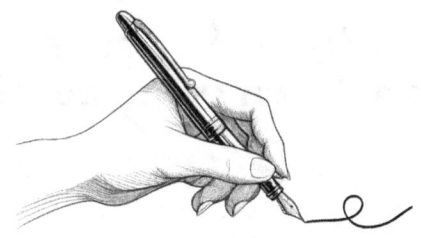

Get Into a Writing Habit Using Dual Expression™.

Start your own practice and use your own voice to spark your own inspiration and seeds of strength. Here are the instructions:

1. Make a recording about items on your mind from your prayer/devotional time, writing prompt, or inspiring thought.

2. Leave it for at least 1 hour.

3. Listen to the recording and write for five minutes about everything you heard, including pauses, tone shifts, and emotions.

4. Dive deeper into that for future growth and inspiration and do the work.

It's just that simple.
And it's just that powerful.

ABOUT THE AUTHOR

TIFFANY VAKILIAN, CEO AND FOUNDER OF SPEAK FIRE PUBLISHING

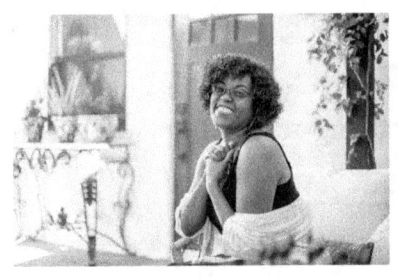 Tiffany Vakilian is an entrepreneur with her Master's (and certification) in Transformative Language Arts. She is also an award-winning poet and performer committed to helping people use spoken, written, sung, or embodied word-art to facilitate social awareness and connection worldwide. Tiffany has a bold, yet tender style about her speaking that unlocks hidden stories within the audience, inspiring people to want to share those stories.

She started SpeakFire Publishing to help unpublished authors go from holding their stories inside to confidently sharing polished, published books on the global stage.

Book to Speak:

Call 619-292-8772 or Email tiffany@speakfirepublishing.com

Great For:
- Keynote
- Conferences
- Church Services
- Women's Retreats

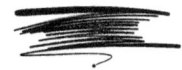

Once you find your people, they will *blow you away* by how long they've been waiting to connect with you **through *your* story**! *Let's talk about what you've learned and how you are moving forward since our breakthrough session.*

Please email me about your progress.

www.speakfirepublishing.com/coaching is where I can coach you as you work on your writing (in small or large sections).

I am also a publisher who can help you with everything from evaluation to editing, formatting, cover design, publishing, and copyright.

Instagram: @tiffanyvakilian
LinkedIn: tiffanyvakilian
Facebook: @TiffanyVakilian
TikTok: @thetiffanyvakilian
Sign up for your FREE Author Breakthrough Session at www.speakfirepublishing.com/

ALSO BY TIFFANY VAKILIAN

The Cry: Poems of Mourning Sickness
https://amzn.to/ 3FBzp7W

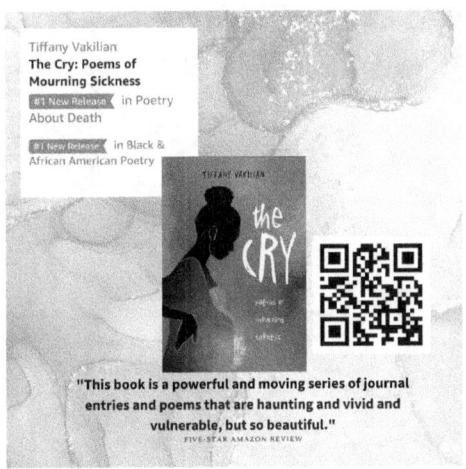

Accountability and Community made my book everything it will ever be.

I wrote this book for women who have experienced infant loss, and for their families and friends, including my son. They were in one or more of my communities, and they were waiting for me to tell my story.

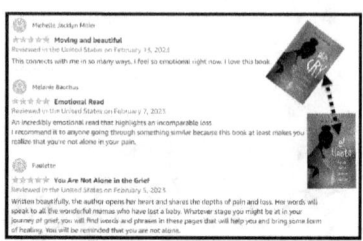

El Llanto: Poemas Sobre el Malestar Matutino
(Spanish Edition) – https://amzn.to/3AP5yc4 eBook

I Need to Stay Faithful, Else Y'all Gonna F.A.A.F.O.
https://amzn.to/3UlZ0FU

Ugly Drawers, Pretty Panties: A Collection of Poetry, Prose, Dreams and Missives https://amzn.to/3NwOz05e

REFERENCES

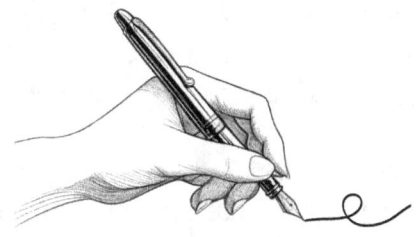

Ambitiously Alexa. (2024, June 6). 40 trauma healing journal prompts to process your past. https://ambitiously alexa.com/trauma-healing-journal-prompts/ (Accessed September 15, 2024)

Day One. (n.d.). Journaling about trauma. https://dayonea pp.com/blog/journaling-about-trauma/ (Accessed September 18, 2024)

Grand Rapids Therapy Group. (n.d.). Journaling: Addressing trauma through writing. https://grandrapidstherapygroup.com/journaling-a ddressing-trauma-through-writing/ (Accessed September 20, 2024)

Errington, H. (n.d.). Creating a safe space for writing. Helen Errington's Newsletter. https://helenerrington.subst ack.com/p/creating-a-safe-space-for-writing (Accessed September 22, 2024)

Friedman, J. (n.d.). You are not your traumas, but here's how to write about them. Jane Fried-

man. https://janefriedman.com/you-are-not-your-tra
umas-but-heres-how-to-write-about-them/ (Accessed
September 25, 2024)

Malibu Mama Loves. (n.d.). 23 journal prompts for processing trauma. https://malibumamaloves.com/23-jou
rnal-prompts-for-processing-trauma/ (Accessed September 27, 2024)

PositivePsychology.com. (n.d.). 83 benefits of journaling
for depression, anxiety, and stress. https://positivepsyc
hology.com/journaling-prompts/ (Accessed September
29, 2024)

Self Heal Journey. (2023, June 17). Journal prompts
for healing. https://selfhealjourney.com/2023/06/17/jou
rnal-prompts-for-healing-2/ (Accessed September 30,
2024)

Choosing Therapy. (n.d.). Journaling about trauma: Benefits & how to get started. https://www.choosingtherapy
.com/journaling-about-trauma/ (Accessed September 5,
2024)

Reddit. (2024). How to begin journaling to cope with
trauma?   r/Journaling.
https://www.reddit.com/r/Journaling/comments/1crs3m
5/how_to_begin_journaling_to_cope_with_trauma/
(Accessed September 10, 2024)

There may be times when the subject matter or poetry may
trigger the pain of a memory or emotional wound. You are
not alone. If you need help, or someone to talk to, here are
some resources to reach out to:

- International Childbirth Association
800-624-4934

- National Resource Center (Parenting/
Relationships) – 800-367-6724

- National Sexual Assault Hotline – 800-656-4673
(available 24 hours)

(available 24 hours)

- National Suicide Prevention Lifeline Available 24/7 at 1-800-273-8255

- You can also reach out for help by texting the word HOME to 741741

- National Women's Health Information Center – 800-994-WOMAN

- M.E.N.D. (Mommies Enduring Neonatal Death) – www.mend.org/virtual-support-group-links

- Parents Helping Parents (free self-help support groups) – 800-882-1250

- Postpartum Support International – 800-944-4773 – www.postpartum.net/get-help/loss-grief-in-pr egnancy-postpartum

- Postpartum Support International – Find Local Support – www.postpartum.net/get-help/locatio ns